COMPLETE GUIDE TO FATTY LIVER DISEASE

A Comprehensive Manual For Diagnosis, Treatment, Prevention, Essential Strategies, Nutritional Insights, Lifestyle Changes, And Herbal Remedies Unveiled

DEHART HAIRSTON

© [DEHART HAIRSTON], [2024]

All rights reserved. No part of this publication may be reproduced, distributed, or transmitted in any form or by any means, including photocopying, recording, or other electronic or mechanical methods, without the prior written permission of the publisher, except in the case of brief quotations embodied in critical reviews and certain other noncommercial uses permitted by copyright law.

DISCLAIMER

This book's content is only intended for general informative purposes. At the time of writing, the author has taken every precaution to guarantee that the material is correct and current. Nevertheless, the author disclaims all explicit and implicit representations and guarantees about the availability, appropriateness, correctness, completeness, and usefulness of the material on these pages.

Since the author is not a licensed medical practitioner, the material in this book shouldn't be interpreted as medical advice. Before making any modifications to their diet, exercise regimen, or medical treatment, readers are urged to speak with a licensed healthcare provider.

Moreover, the author has no connection to any of the businesses, organizations, or people that are discussed in this book. Any mentions of goods, services, businesses, or people are purely informative and do not indicate endorsement or suggestion.

This book's content is entirely dependent on the author's expertise, study, and comprehension of the topic. Despite having taken reasonable care to offer correct information, the author disclaims all liability for any mistakes or omissions in the material as well as for any losses, harm, or damages resulting from using the information.

It is recommended that readers use their own judgment and discretion when applying the knowledge in this book to their own situations. The use or implementation of any material in this book may result in unfavorable repercussions, directly or indirectly, for which the author assumes no liability.

By reading this book, you agree to release and hold the author harmless from any claims, losses, liabilities, costs, or expenditures resulting from or related to the use of the information you get from it.

Table of Contents

CHAPTER 1 13
Introduction To Fatty Liver Disease 13
Understanding The Liver And Its Functions 13
What Is Fatty Liver Disease? 13
Types Of Fatty Liver Disease 14
Causes And Risk Factors 15

CHAPTER 2 17
Signs And Symptoms 17
Identifying Common Symptoms Of Fatty Liver Disease 17
Recognizing When To Seek Medical Help 19
Understanding The Progression Of Symptoms 20

CHAPTER 3 23
Diagnosis 23
Diagnostic Tests And Procedures For Fatty Liver Disease 23
    1. Liver Function Tests (LFTs): 23
    2. Imaging studies: 24
    3. Liver Biopsy: 24
    4. Blood Tests for Metabolic Disorders: 25
    5. Other Tests: 25

Interpretation Of Test Results 25
    1. Liver enzymes: 26
    3. Liver Biopsy Results: 26
    4. Clinical History and Risk Factors: 26
Importance Of Early Detection 27
    1. Complication Prevention: 27
    2. Lifestyle modifications: 27
    3. Monitoring and management: 28
    4. Patient Education and Support: 28
CHAPTER 4 31
Types Of Fatty Liver Disease 31
Non-Alcoholic Fatty Liver Disease (NAFLD) 31
    Understanding NAFLD progression: 31
    Risk Factors and Symptoms: 32
    Management and treatment: 32
Alcoholic Fatty Liver Disease (AFLD) 33
    Understanding AFLD progression: 33
    Risk Factors and Symptoms: 34
    Management and treatment: 34
Key Differences And Similarities 35
CHAPTER 5 37

Complications 37
Potential Complications Associated With Fatty Liver Disease 37
    Liver injury and inflammation 37
    Increased risk of cardiovascular disease 38
    Type II Diabetes and Metabolic Syndrome 38
    Liver cancer 39
    Ascites and edema 39
    Hepatic encephalopathy 40
Impact On Overall Health 41
    Insulin Resistance and Diabetes 41
    Dyslipidemia and CVD 41
    Obesity and Metabolic Syndrome 42
    Psychosocial Impact 43
Long-Term Consequences 43
    Liver failure 43
    Reduced quality of life 44
    Mortality Risk 45
CHAPTER 6 47
Lifestyle Changes And Prevention 47
Dietary Recommendations For Managing Fatty Liver Disease 47

Importance Of Regular Exercise 49
Strategies For Reducing Risk Factors 51
CHAPTER 7 53
Medical Treatments 53
Medications For Fatty Liver Disease 53
Surgical And Non-Surgical Interventions 55
Potential Side Effects And Risks 56
CHAPTER 8 59
Alternative Therapies 59
Role Of Complementary And Alternative Medicine
.... 59
Herbal Supplements And Their Efficacy 61
Consultation With Healthcare Providers 63
CHAPTER 9 67
Living With Fatty Liver Disease 67
Coping Strategies For Managing Symptoms 67
Support Networks And Resources 69
Maintaining A Positive Outlook 71
CHAPTER 10 75
Future Directions And Research 75
Current Advancements In Fatty Liver Disease
Research 75

Promising Treatments On The Horizon 77
Opportunities For Further Study And Awareness 80
CONCLUSION..83
THE END 86

ABOUT THIS BOOK

"Fatty Liver Disease" is more than just another health book; it is a must-read handbook that can change people's lives. In today's society, when lifestyle choices can have an impact on our health, knowing and controlling illnesses such as fatty liver disease is critical. This book is a beacon of information, putting light on a malady that affects millions throughout the globe.

Chapter by chapter, readers are taken on a tour through the complexities of fatty liver disease. It starts with a thorough introduction that demystifies the liver's function and describes the numerous forms, causes, and risk factors linked with the ailment. From then, it digs into the critical parts of signs and symptoms, assisting people in recognizing warning signals and understanding when to seek medical attention.

Another key chapter is Diagnosis, which discusses diagnostic testing, data interpretation, and the need for early diagnosis. Understanding the many forms of fatty liver disease is critical, as explained in Chapter 4, differentiating between non-alcoholic and alcoholic versions and illuminating their intricacies.

Furthermore, this book goes beyond identification, providing readers with information on probable problems, lifestyle changes, medical treatments, and alternative medicines. It provides people with practical information on dietary adjustments, exercise regimens, and preventative measures, giving them hope and agency in managing their health efficiently.

The chapters on living with fatty liver disease and future directions take a comprehensive approach, covering not only the medical but also the emotional and psychological elements of the illness.

By giving coping skills, support networks, and insights into current research, this book serves as a companion on the path to improved health.

Finally, "Fatty Liver Disease" is essential for anybody dealing with this ailment or worried about their liver's health. It serves as a road map for understanding, controlling, and even conquering fatty liver disease, making it an essential resource for anybody looking to take charge of their health.

CHAPTER 1

Introduction To Fatty Liver Disease

Understanding The Liver And Its Functions

The liver, the body's biggest internal organ, is placed directly under the rib cage on the right side of the belly and is sometimes neglected despite its importance to human health. It's like a chemical factory, with over 500 essential tasks that keep us healthy. One of its key functions is to digest everything we eat, including food, drugs, alcohol, and pollutants. It also produces bile, which aids in fat digestion, stores glucose in the form of glycogen for energy, and filters toxic compounds from the blood.

What Is Fatty Liver Disease?

Fatty liver disease, also known as hepatic steatosis, arises when fat accumulates in liver cells and impairs their function. This illness is growing more common, affecting individuals of all ages, genders, and ethnicities. It is often a quiet disorder, with few or no symptoms in its early stages, making it critical to understand the origins, risk factors, and possible consequences.

Types Of Fatty Liver Disease

1. Alcoholic Fatty Liver Disease (AFLD) occurs as a result of heavy alcohol intake over time. The liver metabolizes alcohol, but persistent alcohol use might exceed its capability, resulting in fat buildup.

2. Non-alcoholic fatty Liver Disease (NAFLD) is more frequent and affects those who do not use excessive amounts of alcohol. Instead, it is often associated with obesity, insulin resistance, high blood sugar, and elevated blood fat levels (hyperlipidemia).

Causes And Risk Factors

Numerous variables influence the development of fatty liver disease, ranging from lifestyle decisions to genetic predispositions. Listed below are some frequent causes and risk factors:

- Obesity, especially visceral fat in the belly, raises the risk of NAFLD.

- Insulin resistance causes the body to produce more insulin, leading to fat storage in the liver.

- Type 2 diabetes increases the chance of developing NAFLD owing to insulin resistance and metabolic abnormalities.

- High blood lipid levels (triglycerides and LDL cholesterol) may lead to fat deposition in the liver.

- Metabolic Syndrome: Obesity, high blood pressure, high blood sugar, and abnormal cholesterol levels raise the risk of NAFLD.

- Crash diets and quick weight reduction procedures might release fatty acids from adipose tissue, exceeding the liver's ability to digest them.

- Certain drugs, including corticosteroids, tamoxifen, and methotrexate, might lead to liver fat buildup.

Understanding these causes and risk factors is critical for developing preventative and therapy strategies for fatty liver disease. Individuals may prevent liver disease by treating underlying concerns such as obesity, diabetes, and lifestyle behaviors.

CHAPTER 2

Signs And Symptoms

Identifying Common Symptoms Of Fatty Liver Disease

Fatty liver disease often causes a variety of symptoms, although other people may have none at all, particularly in the early stages. One of the most prevalent symptoms is exhaustion, which might present as a general feeling of tiredness or weakness. This weariness may remain after enough rest, affecting daily activities and general quality of life.

Another noticeable sign is stomach discomfort or pain, which is usually seen in the upper right quadrant, where the liver is located. This pain may range in severity from moderate to severe, and it may be accompanied by bloating or a sense of fullness. Some people report feeling nauseous or vomiting after eating fatty or oily meals.

In addition, those with fatty liver disease may have unexplained weight loss or lack of appetite. This might be due to a variety of reasons, including changes in metabolism and reduced food absorption by the liver. In contrast, some people may gain weight, especially in the abdomen, which may worsen pre-existing symptoms and raise the risk of problems.

Other warning signs include jaundice, which causes yellowing of the skin and eyes, as well as black urine. These symptoms suggest compromised liver function and need rapid medical treatment. It's crucial to remember that not everyone with fatty liver disease may have all of these symptoms, and others may just have moderate or vague indicators.

Recognizing When To Seek Medical Help

Understanding when to seek medical attention is critical for properly treating fatty liver disease. If you are experiencing chronic exhaustion, stomach discomfort, or any of the other symptoms listed above, you should see a healthcare expert right away. Furthermore, if you see any symptoms of jaundice, such as yellowing of the skin or eyes, get medical assistance right once, since this might suggest significant liver damage.

Furthermore, if you already have risk factors for fatty liver disease, such as obesity, diabetes, or high cholesterol, you should have frequent screening tests to evaluate your liver health. These tests may include blood tests to examine liver function as well as imaging procedures like ultrasounds or MRI scans to determine the amount of liver damage.

In certain circumstances, fatty liver disease may lead to more serious problems such as liver fibrosis, cirrhosis, or cancer. As a result, early identification and care are critical for avoiding severe consequences and maintaining liver function. Your healthcare professional might suggest suitable lifestyle modifications, medicines, or other measures to assist manage the illness and avoid future liver damage.

Understanding The Progression Of Symptoms

The course of symptoms in fatty liver disease varies greatly based on many variables, including the underlying etiology, the individual's general health, and lifestyle choices. Many persons with fatty liver disease may not exhibit any visible symptoms in its early stages, making detection difficult.

As fatty liver disease advances, tiredness, stomach discomfort, and nausea may worsen. This is often symptomatic of declining liver function and increased inflammation inside the liver tissue. If left untreated, fatty liver disease may proceed to more severe stages such as liver fibrosis and cirrhosis, both of which cause permanent scarring of the liver tissue.

In certain situations, fatty liver disease may raise the chance of developing other major health problems, including cardiovascular disease, type 2 diabetes, and liver cancer. As a result, it is critical to regularly monitor symptoms and get medical assistance if you notice any unusual changes in your health.

Understanding the evolution of symptoms associated with fatty liver disease allows patients to make proactive efforts to successfully manage the illness and limit the risk of consequences. This might include leading a healthy lifestyle that includes regular exercise, a balanced diet, and avoiding alcohol and other liver-damaging chemicals. Furthermore, collaborating with healthcare experts to monitor liver health and treat any underlying risk factors may help avoid the advancement of fatty liver disease and improve overall health outcomes.

CHAPTER 3

Diagnosis

Diagnostic Tests And Procedures For Fatty Liver Disease

When diagnosing fatty liver disease, healthcare experts use several tests and procedures to get a thorough picture of the issue. These tests aid in evaluating the severity of liver damage and directing suitable treatment methods.

1. Liver Function Tests (LFTs): These blood tests measure the amounts of enzymes and proteins generated by the liver. Elevated levels of enzymes like ALT (alanine transaminase) and AST (aspartate transaminase) might suggest liver inflammation and injury.

2. Imaging studies:

- Ultrasound creates pictures of the liver using sound waves. It may identify fatty infiltration and evaluate liver size and texture.

- CT Scan or MRI: These imaging procedures give comprehensive images of the liver, allowing for evaluation of fatty deposits and accompanying problems.

- Transient Elastography (FibroScan): A non-invasive technique that detects liver stiffness and fibrosis.

3. Liver Biopsy: In certain situations, a liver biopsy may be required to confirm the diagnosis and determine the extent of liver damage. During this process, a tiny tissue sample from the liver is collected and analyzed under a microscope.

4. **Blood Tests for Metabolic Disorders:** Because fatty liver disease is often related to disorders like obesity, diabetes, and high cholesterol, blood tests to assess these metabolic variables may be conducted to determine the underlying cause.

5. **Other Tests:** Depending on the circumstances, further tests such as viral hepatitis screening, genetic testing for hereditary liver illnesses, and tests for autoimmune liver diseases may be performed.

Interpretation Of Test Results

Interpreting diagnostic test findings for fatty liver disease requires thorough examination and consideration of many aspects. Elevated liver enzyme levels, fatty infiltration on imaging investigations, and biopsy results are all significant signs.

1. **Liver enzymes:** Elevated levels of ALT and AST indicate liver inflammation and damage. However, it's crucial to remember that these enzymes may be increased in illnesses unrelated to the liver, so further testing is required.

2. Ultrasound, CT scans, and MRI may detect fatty deposits in the liver and determine the extent of liver damage. The level of steatosis (fat buildup) and any evidence of liver damage or consequences are assessed.

3. **Liver Biopsy Results:** A liver biopsy is the most reliable way to examine liver health because it allows for direct imaging of liver tissue under a microscope. It aids in the detection and amount of steatosis, inflammation, fibrosis, and other liver disorders.

4. **Clinical History and Risk Factors:** Understanding a patient's medical history, including risk factors

including obesity, diabetes, alcohol usage, and a family history of liver disease, is critical for effective diagnosis and treatment.

Importance Of Early Detection

Early identification of fatty liver disease is critical to limiting disease progression and consequences. By detecting the illness early on, healthcare practitioners may conduct therapies to prevent or cure liver damage and enhance long-term results.

1. Complication Prevention: If fatty liver disease is not treated, it may proceed to more serious illnesses such as non-alcoholic steatohepatitis (NASH), cirrhosis, liver failure, and hepatocellular carcinoma. Early identification enables early management to avoid these consequences.

2. Lifestyle modifications: Early diagnosis allows patients to make the required lifestyle modifications to promote liver health.

This involves eating a nutritious diet, staying in a healthy weight range, exercising frequently, minimizing alcohol intake, and addressing underlying illnesses like diabetes and high cholesterol.

3. **Monitoring and management:** Individuals with fatty liver disease need regular monitoring of liver function and disease development. Early detection allows healthcare practitioners to carefully follow patients and alter treatment procedures as necessary to improve results.

4. **Patient Education and Support:** An early diagnosis enables proactive patient education regarding the significance of liver health, the relevance of lifestyle changes, and the possible consequences of untreated fatty liver disease. Empowering patients with information and assistance may help them stick to treatment programs and improve their overall health.

In conclusion, rapid detection of fatty liver disease using suitable diagnostic tests and methods is crucial for commencing early management, avoiding complications, and improving patient outcomes. Healthcare personnel are critical in detecting the signs and symptoms of fatty liver disease, providing thorough assessments, and advising patients on appropriate treatment measures.

CHAPTER 4

Types Of Fatty Liver Disease

Non-Alcoholic Fatty Liver Disease (NAFLD)

Non-alcoholic fatty liver disease (NAFLD) is a common illness in which fat accumulates in the liver but is not caused by excessive alcohol intake. It is often linked to obesity, insulin resistance, high blood sugar, and excessive quantities of fat in the blood. NAFLD usually proceeds through multiple phases, beginning with simple fatty liver (steatosis) and perhaps progressing to non-alcoholic steatohepatitis (NASH), fibrosis, and cirrhosis.

Understanding NAFLD progression:

NAFLD begins with the buildup of fat in liver cells, which may cause inflammation and damage over time. In certain instances, this inflammation develops into NASH, which causes liver cell destruction and scarring, decreasing liver function. If left untreated, NASH may progress to fibrosis, which occurs when scar tissue replaces good liver tissue, and eventually to cirrhosis, a severe disease in which the liver is permanently destroyed.

Risk Factors and Symptoms:

Obesity, type 2 diabetes, high cholesterol, metabolic syndrome, and certain drugs all increase the risk of developing NAFLD. Symptoms are often nonexistent in the early stages, although they may include tiredness, weakness, stomach discomfort, and an enlarged liver. Blood tests, imaging examinations (such as ultrasound or MRI), and, on occasion, a liver biopsy are used to make the diagnosis.

Management and treatment:

The treatment for NAFLD focuses on addressing underlying risk factors and avoiding disease development.

This involves lifestyle changes including weight reduction, frequent exercise, and a nutritious diet low in sugar and saturated fats. Medications may be recommended to treat diabetes, excessive cholesterol, or liver inflammation.

Alcoholic Fatty Liver Disease (AFLD)

Excessive alcohol intake causes alcoholic fatty liver disease (AFLD), which is one of the early phases of alcohol-related liver disease. AFLD, like NAFLD, is caused by fat buildup in liver cells, but it is specifically connected to alcohol use. If alcohol usage persists, AFLD may lead to more serious illnesses such as alcoholic hepatitis and cirrhosis.

Understanding AFLD progression:

Excessive alcohol intake impairs the liver's capacity to adequately metabolize alcohol, resulting in fat buildup in liver cells. This may eventually lead to inflammation and liver tissue damage.

With chronic alcohol usage, AFLD may proceed to alcoholic hepatitis, which is marked by liver inflammation and possibly fatal consequences. In rare instances, AFLD may proceed to cirrhosis, which causes significant scarring and affects liver function.

Risk Factors and Symptoms:

The major risk factor for AFLD is excessive alcohol drinking, however individual susceptibility varies. Symptoms might include stomach discomfort, exhaustion, jaundice (yellowing of the skin and eyes), and swelling in the belly or legs. Medical history, physical examination, blood tests, imaging scans, and, in certain cases, a liver biopsy are used to make the diagnosis.

Management and treatment:

The most effective therapy for AFLD is to avoid consuming alcohol. For those with moderate AFLD, refraining from alcohol may frequently reverse liver damage. However, for patients with severe illnesses or consequences, like as cirrhosis, more medical care may be required. This may involve symptom-management drugs, dietary assistance, and, in extreme situations, liver transplants.

Key Differences And Similarities

While NAFLD and AFLD both involve fat buildup in the liver, the underlying reasons are quite different. NAFLD is connected to metabolic disorders including obesity and insulin resistance, while AFLD is directly related to alcohol usage. If left untreated, these disorders might lead to more serious liver disease.

Despite their separate etiologies, NAFLD and AFLD have comparable development and treatment patterns. Both disorders may cause liver damage at various stages, including inflammation, fibrosis, and cirrhosis. Similarly, the cornerstone of therapy for both NAFLD and AFLD is treating underlying risk factors and encouraging liver health via lifestyle changes including diet and exercise.

Understanding the distinctions and similarities between NAFLD and AFLD is critical for proper diagnosis and treatment. By diagnosing the underlying cause of fatty liver disease and applying focused therapies, healthcare practitioners may help patients manage their condition and decrease the risk of complications.

CHAPTER 5

Complications

Potential Complications Associated With Fatty Liver Disease

While fatty liver disease may seem to be harmless at first, it may quickly escalate into a series of consequences if not treated. Understanding these possible problems is critical for treating the disease successfully.

Liver injury and inflammation

As fatty liver disease worsens, it may cause inflammation and damage to liver cells. This inflammation may result in a disorder known as non-alcoholic steatohepatitis (NASH), which is marked by liver cell damage and inflammation. NASH may proceed to fibrosis, which is when scar tissue accumulates in the liver.

In extreme situations, this fibrosis may lead to cirrhosis, which occurs when the liver becomes badly damaged and loses its capacity to function correctly.

Increased risk of cardiovascular disease

Individuals with fatty liver disease have a higher chance of acquiring cardiovascular disease. Fat buildup in the liver is often associated with a rise in triglyceride and other lipid levels in the blood, which may contribute to atherosclerosis. This increases the likelihood of a heart attack, stroke, and other cardiovascular issues.

Type II Diabetes and Metabolic Syndrome

Fatty liver disease is strongly associated with insulin resistance, a condition in which the body's cells become less receptive to insulin. Insulin resistance is characteristic of type 2 diabetes and metabolic syndrome, both of which are linked to fatty liver disease. The presence of these disorders may worsen liver damage and raise the risk of consequences.

Liver cancer

In the late stages of fatty liver disease, especially cirrhosis, there is an increased chance of developing liver cancer, commonly known as hepatocellular carcinoma (HCC). Chronic inflammation and liver cell damage lead to the growth of malignant tumors in the liver. Regular monitoring and early intervention are critical for detecting and treating liver cancer in its early stages.

Ascites and edema

Cirrhosis, a severe consequence of fatty liver disease, may cause fluid accumulation in the abdomen, also known as ascites. Ascites are caused by increased pressure in the blood arteries around the liver, which allows fluid to flow into the abdominal cavity. This may lead to stomach swelling, pain, and trouble breathing. Edema, or swelling in the legs and feet, may also result from reduced liver function and blood flow alterations.

Hepatic encephalopathy

In the latter stages of liver disease, notably cirrhosis, the liver's capacity to metabolize toxic compounds is compromised. This may result in the buildup of poisons in the circulation, such as ammonia. Hepatic encephalopathy develops when these poisons disrupt brain function, causing disorientation, cognitive impairment, and, in extreme instances, coma. Management techniques try to minimize toxin accumulation and enhance liver function to relieve symptoms.

Impact On Overall Health

Fatty liver disease affects not just the liver but also the rest of the body. The interaction of liver function, metabolism, and inflammation may affect several organ systems, resulting in a variety of health concerns.

Insulin Resistance and Diabetes

Insulin resistance, a typical characteristic of fatty liver disease, may lead to type 2 diabetes. The liver regulates blood sugar levels by storing and releasing glucose as required. When the liver becomes insulin resistant, it overproduces glucose, causing high blood sugar levels. This may eventually lead to diabetes and its consequences, such as cardiovascular disease and nerve damage.

Dyslipidemia and CVD

Fatty liver disease is often related to dyslipidemia, which is defined by high levels of triglycerides and

LDL cholesterol and low levels of HDL. These lipid abnormalities may contribute to the development of atherosclerosis, raising the risk of heart attacks and strokes. Managing lipid levels with lifestyle changes and medicines is critical for lowering cardiovascular risk in people with fatty liver disease.

Obesity and Metabolic Syndrome

Obesity is a significant risk factor for fatty liver disease, and the two illnesses often coexist. Excess fat, especially visceral fat around the belly, leads to insulin resistance, inflammation, and dyslipidemia, which are generally referred to as metabolic syndrome. Metabolic syndrome heightens the risk of cardiovascular disease, type 2 diabetes, and fatty liver disease development. Weight reduction and lifestyle improvements are critical components in treating obesity and fatty liver disease.

Psychosocial Impact

Living with a chronic ailment, such as fatty liver disease, may hurt mental and emotional health. The ambiguity around the disease's course, the need for lifestyle changes, and possible consequences may cause worry, despair, and a worse quality of life. Building a support network, seeking counseling or therapy, and participating in stress-reduction activities may all help people deal with the psychological aspects of treating fatty liver disease.

Long-Term Consequences

The long-term effects of fatty liver disease highlight the need for early identification, intervention, and continued care to avoid progression and reduce risks.

Liver failure

Liver failure is possible in severe instances of fatty liver disease, especially when combined with cirrhosis. Liver failure is a life-threatening illness in which the liver loses its capacity to conduct vital tasks such as detoxification, protein synthesis, and bile generation. This may cause a series of problems, including jaundice, hepatic encephalopathy, and fluid retention, demanding immediate medical attention, such as liver transplantation.

Reduced quality of life

Chronic liver disease may have a major effect on quality of life owing to symptoms including weariness, stomach pain, and cognitive impairment. The stress of managing the condition, following treatment plans, and dealing with possible consequences may all have an impact on emotional well-being and social functioning. Multidisciplinary care techniques that address physical, emotional, and social needs may enhance the quality of life for people with fatty liver disease.

Mortality Risk

Fatty liver disease is connected with an increased risk of death, especially in instances of severe liver fibrosis, cirrhosis, and liver cancer. Complications such as liver failure, cardiovascular events, and hepatocellular carcinoma may drastically reduce life expectancy if not properly controlled. Early detection, risk stratification, and prompt therapies are critical for lowering mortality risk and improving long-term outcomes in people with fatty liver disease.

CHAPTER 6

Lifestyle Changes And Prevention

Dietary Recommendations For Managing Fatty Liver Disease

Diet is an important factor in controlling fatty liver disease. Making wise dietary choices may considerably enhance liver health and minimize the chance of problems. A balanced diet reduced in saturated fats, refined carbohydrates, and processed foods is essential. Instead, try to include lots of fruits, veggies, nutritious grains, and lean meats in your meals.

One of the most significant dietary suggestions for controlling fatty liver disease is to reduce your consumption of added sugars and high-fructose corn syrup. These components are widely found in sugary beverages such as soda, fruit juices, and sports drinks, as well as in many packaged meals.

Consuming too much sugar may cause fat storage in the liver, worsening the illness. Instead, satisfy your thirst with water, herbal teas, or naturally flavored sparkling water.

Another dietary recommendation is to choose healthy fats over harmful ones. While saturated and trans fats in fried meals, fatty meats, and baked products may cause liver inflammation and damage, unsaturated fats in avocados, nuts, seeds, and olive oil can protect the liver. Including these healthy fats in your diet may help to decrease inflammation and enhance liver function.

It's also vital to control your portion sizes and total calorie consumption. Consuming more calories than your body requires may cause weight gain, which is a significant risk factor for fatty liver disease. Portion management and attention to hunger and fullness signals may help you balance your calorie intake and maintain a healthy weight.

Importance Of Regular Exercise

In addition to dietary adjustments, frequent exercise is an important part of controlling fatty liver disease. Physical exercise provides various advantages for liver health, including fat loss, improved insulin sensitivity, and reduced inflammation. Aim for 30 minutes of moderate-intensity activity most days of the week, such as brisk walking, cycling, swimming, or dancing.

Exercise not only helps with weight control, but it also has a direct impact on liver function. When you exercise, your muscles utilize glucose for energy, lowering blood sugar levels and reducing the amount of sugar deposited in the liver as fat. Furthermore, exercise increases the synthesis of enzymes that aid in the breakdown of fat in the liver, resulting in a decrease in liver fat buildup over time.

In addition to cardiovascular activity, including strength training in your program might be advantageous. Building muscle mass not only boosts your metabolism, allowing you to burn more calories at rest, but it also improves insulin sensitivity and lowers liver fat. Aim to include resistance training activities, such as weightlifting or bodyweight exercises, at least twice a week.

Making exercise a regular part of your routine might be difficult at first, but finding things you love and implementing them into your daily schedule will help you stay with it in the long run. Whether it's going for a stroll with a buddy, taking a dancing class, or joining a sports team, finding methods to keep active that you love is essential for sticking to a regular fitness regimen.

Strategies For Reducing Risk Factors

In addition to dietary adjustments and regular exercise, you may use a variety of different measures to minimize your chance of developing fatty liver. One of the most crucial is to keep a healthy weight. Excess body weight, particularly around the belly, is closely linked to an elevated risk of fatty liver disease and related consequences. Even a little drop of weight may have a major influence on liver function, so strive for steady, long-term weight loss via a mix of food, exercise, and lifestyle modifications.

Another significant risk element to consider is alcohol usage. Excess alcohol use is a primary cause of liver damage and may worsen fatty liver disease. If you have fatty liver disease, you should reduce your alcohol use or, preferably, avoid alcohol completely.

Consult your healthcare professional if you need assistance or resources to help you limit your alcohol consumption.

In addition to keeping a healthy weight and reducing alcohol intake, it's critical to address other underlying health issues that might lead to fatty liver disease, such as high cholesterol, high blood pressure, and type 2 diabetes. Working with your healthcare professional to address these problems via medication, lifestyle modifications, and frequent monitoring may help to lessen the pressure on your liver and the risk of consequences.

Finally, living a healthy lifestyle may help minimize your chance of developing fatty liver disease while also improving your overall health and well-being. This includes getting adequate sleep, reducing stress, quitting smoking, and keeping hydrated.

CHAPTER 7

Medical Treatments

Medications For Fatty Liver Disease

Medications are essential in the management of fatty liver disease, to relieve symptoms, reduce liver inflammation, and prevent consequences. While there is no one medicine intended to treat fatty liver disease, physicians often prescribe medications to address underlying disorders that contribute to its development, such as diabetes, high cholesterol, or obesity.

Pioglitazone is a regularly given medicine that improves insulin sensitivity and reduces liver inflammation. Pioglitazone improves insulin activity, which helps manage blood sugar levels and may decrease the onset of fatty liver.

However, it is critical to watch for possible adverse effects such as weight gain and fluid retention.

Another often-used drug is vitamin E, which is recognized for its antioxidant effects. Antioxidants prevent oxidative stress, which is a major cause of liver damage. Vitamin E supplementation has shown promise in lowering liver inflammation and may help certain people with nonalcoholic fatty liver disease (NAFLD). Nonetheless, its efficacy varies, and it is not appropriate for everyone, especially those with certain medical problems or using certain drugs.

Doctors may also prescribe statins to regulate cholesterol levels and lower the risk of cardiovascular disease, which is usually associated with fatty liver disease. Statins function by suppressing cholesterol formation in the liver, which lowers blood cholesterol levels. While statins are typically safe, they might induce adverse effects such as muscular discomfort or abnormal liver enzyme levels, necessitating constant monitoring.

Surgical And Non-Surgical Interventions

In extreme situations of fatty liver disease, when lifestyle modifications and medicines are insufficient, surgical and non-surgical procedures may be explored to treat complications or advanced liver damage.

Liver transplantation is the only therapy for end-stage liver disease, including cirrhosis caused by advanced non-alcoholic steatohepatitis (NASH). During a liver transplant, a damaged liver is replaced with a healthy donor liver. Individuals with severe liver dysfunction may be able to survive and have a higher quality of life after undergoing this treatment.

Non-surgical therapies include bariatric surgery for those suffering from obesity-related fatty liver disease. Bariatric surgery seeks to lose weight by lowering stomach size or rerouting the digestive system, resulting in considerable improvements in liver function and metabolic parameters. However, it is critical to do a complete study to verify eligibility and weigh possible risks and advantages.

Potential Side Effects And Risks

While drugs and therapies provide therapeutic advantages, they also have possible side effects and hazards that must be carefully considered and monitored.

Common adverse effects of fatty liver disease treatments include gastrointestinal issues, migraines, and muscular discomfort. Patients should quickly report any adverse reactions to their healthcare practitioner so that therapy may be adjusted as needed.

Furthermore, certain drugs may interfere with other prescriptions or underlying medical issues, highlighting the significance of a thorough medical examination and monitoring.

Surgical procedures, such as liver transplantation or bariatric surgery, include inherent risks, including surgical complications, infections, and organ rejection (in the case of transplantation). Patients having these treatments need a complete pre-operative evaluation, post-operative care, and long-term follow-up to maximize results and reduce problems.

Finally, although medicinal therapies may help manage fatty liver disease, they must be approached with caution, taking into account specific patient variables, possible advantages, and dangers.

CHAPTER 8

Alternative Therapies

Role Of Complementary And Alternative Medicine

When it comes to controlling fatty liver disease, complementary and alternative medicine (CAM) may provide additional options to traditional therapies. CAM refers to a broad variety of activities and treatments that are beyond the scope of orthodox medicine. These may include acupuncture, herbal medicines, nutritional supplements, meditation, and yoga, among others.

One of the primary responsibilities of complementary and alternative medicine (CAM) in the treatment of fatty liver disease is to promote holistic recovery. CAM techniques often emphasize treating the whole person rather than simply the symptoms. This might include lifestyle adjustments, stress-reduction tactics, and nutritional changes designed to promote general well-being and liver health.

For example, acupuncture, an ancient Chinese therapy, involves putting small needles into particular places on the body to promote energy flow. Some research suggests that acupuncture may help decrease liver inflammation and improve liver function in people with fatty liver disease. Similarly, yoga and meditation approaches may help decrease stress, which may promote liver function by decreasing inflammation and boosting relaxation.

However, before incorporating CAM methods into your treatment plan, you should exercise caution and check with your healthcare physician. While many CAM treatments are typically harmless, some may interfere with drugs or worsen existing health concerns.

Furthermore, not all CAM modalities have been well explored for their efficacy in treating fatty liver disease, so it's critical to depend on evidence-based methods and address any possible dangers with your medical team.

Herbal Supplements And Their Efficacy

Herbal supplements have received a lot of interest as prospective treatments for fatty liver disease because of their natural origins and perceived safety. Several herbs and botanical extracts have been investigated for their possible hepatoprotective properties, which means they may help protect the liver from harm and facilitate recovery.

Milk thistle is one of the best-researched herbal treatments for fatty liver disease. Milk thistle includes silymarin, a substance with antioxidant and anti-inflammatory effects.

Some study indicates that silymarin may help decrease liver inflammation, preserve liver cells from injury, and enhance liver function in people with fatty liver disease. However, further high-quality clinical studies are required to validate these results and identify the best dose and duration of therapy.

Turmeric is another plant that shows potential for liver health. Curcumin, the main component in turmeric, has antioxidant and anti-inflammatory qualities that may help people with fatty liver disease. According to studies, curcumin administration may help reduce liver fat buildup, enhance insulin sensitivity, and lower indicators of liver inflammation and fibrosis. Adding turmeric to your diet or taking curcumin supplements under the supervision of a healthcare expert may have potential advantages for treating fatty liver disease.

Dandelion root, artichoke extract, and green tea extract are three other herbal supplements that have been investigated for their possible hepatoprotective properties. While early research indicates encouraging outcomes, further thorough studies are required to determine the safety and effectiveness of these herbal treatments for fatty liver disease. When using herbal supplements, take caution and speak with your healthcare professional to verify they are safe and suitable for your specific requirements.

Consultation With Healthcare Providers

When navigating the complications of fatty liver disease and considering treatment choices, consulting with healthcare experts is critical for customized care and educated decision-making. Healthcare professionals such as primary care doctors, hepatologists, dietitians, and alternative medicine practitioners play critical roles in helping patients through their treatment path and addressing their specific needs and concerns.

Individuals with fatty liver disease may anticipate a thorough evaluation of their medical history, lifestyle variables, and present symptoms when they see a doctor. Healthcare practitioners may arrange diagnostic procedures such as liver function tests, imaging investigations, and liver biopsies to determine the degree of liver damage and modify therapy recommendations appropriately.

In addition to traditional medical treatments, healthcare clinicians may recommend lifestyle adjustments such as dietary changes, exercise routines, weight loss techniques, and alcohol abstinence to enhance liver health and control underlying risk factors for fatty liver disease. They may also advise on pharmaceutical management, including the use of statins, insulin sensitizers, and other pharmacological treatments to treat related illnesses such as dyslipidemia, diabetes, and metabolic syndrome.

Furthermore, persons interested in CAM techniques should talk freely with their healthcare practitioners to ensure safe and coordinated treatment. Healthcare practitioners may advise on evidence-based CAM modalities, their risks and benefits, and potential interactions with conventional therapies. Individuals with fatty liver disease may improve their health outcomes and quality of life by working with healthcare specialists and implementing a multidisciplinary treatment plan.

CHAPTER 9

Living With Fatty Liver Disease

Coping Strategies For Managing Symptoms

Living with fatty liver disease presents several problems, but there are coping methods available to assist manage its symptoms successfully. One of the first stages is to live a healthy lifestyle, which includes eating a well-balanced diet and getting enough exercise. A diet high in fruits, vegetables, lean meats, and whole grains may improve liver function by minimizing fat formation and encouraging weight reduction.

Furthermore, it is critical to minimize consumption of foods heavy in saturated fats, sweets, and processed carbohydrates, since they might accelerate liver damage.

Monitoring portion sizes and practicing mindful eating may also help with weight management and general well-being.

Regular exercise is another important part of controlling fatty liver disease. Physical exercise not only aids in weight control but also increases insulin sensitivity and decreases inflammation, all of which are helpful to liver function. Aim for 30 minutes of moderate-intensity activity most days of the week, such as brisk walking, swimming, or cycling.

Furthermore, regulating stress is critical to maintaining liver function. Chronic stress may exacerbate inflammation and the symptoms of fatty liver disease. Meditation, yoga, deep breathing techniques, and spending time in nature may all help reduce stress.

It is also critical to follow any prescription drugs or therapies indicated by your healthcare practitioner.

These may include drugs to treat underlying illnesses like diabetes, high cholesterol, or hypertension, which may all contribute to liver damage.

Regular monitoring of liver function via blood tests and imaging investigations is critical for following disease development and making necessary therapy adjustments. Maintaining open contact with your healthcare team and following their advice will aid in the effective treatment of fatty liver disease and reduce complications.

Support Networks And Resources

Living with fatty liver disease might be stressful at times, but you don't have to face it alone. Creating a strong support network may give important emotional and practical help during your journey.

Family and friends may be a source of support and understanding, providing a listening ear and a helping hand when necessary. Sharing your experiences with loved ones might help you feel more connected and less alone.

Joining support groups or online forums focused on fatty liver disease may also be quite useful. These forums allow you to connect with people who are going through similar situations, offer advice, and discuss coping tactics. Hearing from those who have effectively controlled their disease may be uplifting and inspiring.

Additionally, consulting with healthcare specialists who specialize in liver health, such as hepatologists or dietitians, may give helpful knowledge and resources targeted to your specific requirements. They may provide professional advice on how to manage symptoms, make lifestyle changes, and seek appropriate medical treatment.

Exploring educational resources such as books, websites, and trustworthy health organizations will help you better understand fatty liver disease and empower you to take charge of your health. Knowledge is a great tool for managing chronic diseases, and remaining educated may help you make better choices about your treatment.

Remember that you are not alone in your journey with fatty liver disease. By seeking assistance and using available services, you may better manage the hurdles and enhance your overall quality of life.

Maintaining A Positive Outlook

While living with fatty liver disease might be difficult, keeping a happy attitude can have a big impact on your overall health. Cultivating a resilient and optimistic mentality can help you deal with the ups and downs of managing the disease.

Concentrate on the areas of your life that you can control, such as living a healthy lifestyle, adhering to your treatment plan, and getting help when necessary. Celebrate little triumphs along the road, such as adhering to a healthy diet, meeting a fitness goal, or improving liver function.

Practice self-compassion and kindness to yourself, acknowledging that treating a chronic disease requires time and effort. Be patient with yourself when you face trials and failures.

Engage in things that provide you pleasure and contentment, such as pursuing hobbies, spending time with loved ones, or discovering new interests. Cultivating a sense of purpose and meaning outside of your condition might help you feel more normal and satisfied in life.

Maintain contact with your support network, relying on loved ones and medical experts for encouragement and advice. Building good connections and cultivating a sense of community may give vital emotional support as you progress.

Finally, be optimistic about the future and the potential for better health and well-being. With effort, persistence, and a positive attitude, you may successfully control fatty liver disease while still living a satisfying lifestyle.

74

CHAPTER 10

Future Directions And Research

Current Advancements In Fatty Liver Disease Research

In recent years, the subject of fatty liver disease study has made considerable advances, thanks to greater awareness and financing. Researchers are diving deeper into the complicated processes that drive the development and evolution of this common illness. One major area of improvement has been the knowledge of the involvement of genetic predispositions, lifestyle variables, and environmental effects in the etiology of fatty liver disease.

Furthermore, technological advancements have transformed diagnostic tools, allowing healthcare practitioners to diagnose fatty liver disease in its early stages with higher precision. Advanced imaging techniques, such as magnetic resonance imaging (MRI) and transient elastography, have emerged as useful tools for non-invasive evaluation of liver fat content and fibrosis development, allowing for prompt intervention and tailored treatment regimens.

Furthermore, the development of high-throughput omics tools such as genomics, transcriptomics, proteomics, and metabolomics has transformed our capacity to understand the intricate molecular networks that underpin fatty liver disease. These cutting-edge techniques have identified new biomarkers and therapeutic targets, opening the path for precision medicine approaches customized to specific patient profiles.

Collaborative research activities at the national and international levels have allowed data exchange and integration, hastening the speed of discovery in fatty liver disease. By encouraging multidisciplinary cooperation among doctors, scientists, and industry partners, researchers are combining their skills to address the numerous problems faced by this global health burden.

In conclusion, contemporary advances in fatty liver disease research use a diverse strategy that combines genetics, technology, and collaborative efforts. These fascinating breakthroughs have the potential to open new insights into disease pathophysiology, improve diagnostic accuracy, and eventually revolutionize treatment techniques for patients globally.

Promising Treatments On The Horizon

The landscape of fatty liver disease therapy is fast changing, with a large pipeline of intriguing therapeutic options on the way. Researchers are looking at a variety of approaches to target the underlying processes that cause liver fat buildup and inflammation, including lifestyle changes, pharmaceutical drugs, and new biologics.

One of the most well-researched therapies is lifestyle modification, which includes dietary adjustments, frequent exercise, and weight control. Clinical studies have shown that organized lifestyle treatments may reduce hepatic steatosis, improve insulin sensitivity, and reduce liver inflammation in people with fatty liver disease. These results emphasize the critical relevance of lifestyle variables in illness management, as well as the value of holistic treatment methods.

In addition to lifestyle changes, pharmaceutical treatments that target critical processes implicated in the etiology of fatty liver disease are being studied. These include insulin sensitizers like thiazolidinediones and glucagon-like peptide-1 receptor agonists, which have shown promise in treating hepatic steatosis and inflammation. Other pharmacological drugs that target lipid metabolism, oxidative stress, and inflammation are also being investigated, potentially providing new therapeutic options for individuals with fatty liver disease.

Furthermore, the science of regenerative medicine has the potential to revolutionize therapies for fatty liver disease. Stem cell therapy, liver transplantation, and tissue engineering methods are being investigated as possible options for restoring liver function and reversing fibrosis in the late stages of the illness. While still in the early phases, these regenerative medicines provide hope to patients with severe liver damage and few therapeutic alternatives.

In summary, potential treatments for fatty liver disease include a wide range of interventions, from lifestyle changes to pharmaceutical agents and regenerative therapies.

By leveraging the power of transdisciplinary research and innovation, physicians and scientists have the potential to revolutionize the landscape of fatty liver disease care and enhance patient outcomes globally.

Opportunities For Further Study And Awareness

Despite substantial advances in research and clinical therapy, there are still various avenues for future investigation and awareness in the area of fatty liver disease. One critical need is to better understand the natural history and long-term effects of fatty liver disease in varied patient groups. Prospective cohort studies and longitudinal registries are critical for monitoring disease development, discovering prognostic indicators, and improving risk stratification tools.

Furthermore, there is an urgent need to raise awareness and early diagnosis of fatty liver disease among healthcare practitioners and the general public. Educational campaigns aimed at primary care doctors, specialists, and the general public may assist promote knowledge of the risk factors, symptoms, and consequences of fatty liver disease, allowing people to seek prompt medical examination and treatment.

Furthermore, differences in access to care and treatment results highlight the necessity of tackling socioeconomic and healthcare inequities in the management of fatty liver disease. Outreach programs, community-based therapies, and legislative measures targeted at increasing healthcare access and equality have the potential to significantly reduce the burden of fatty liver disease on disadvantaged communities.

Furthermore, there is an increasing knowledge of the link between fatty liver disease and other metabolic and cardiovascular disorders, such as obesity, diabetes, and heart disease. More study is required to better understand the intricate relationships between these comorbidities, discover similar pathophysiological mechanisms, and create integrated care methods to meet the overall requirements of patients with metabolic-associated fatty liver disease.

In conclusion, options for additional study and awareness of fatty liver disease include a wide range of research, education, and advocacy projects. By tackling these difficulties front-on, healthcare professionals, academics, policymakers, and community stakeholders may collaborate to expand our knowledge of the illness, improve clinical outcomes, and eventually lessen the worldwide burden of fatty liver disease.

CONCLUSION

To summarize, Fatty Liver Disease (FLD) is a major worldwide health issue owing to its rising prevalence and associated implications. The multifaceted character of FLD, which includes lifestyle variables, genetic predispositions, and metabolic abnormalities, emphasizes the significance of a comprehensive approach to its treatment and prevention.

This investigation demonstrates that early identification and treatments are critical in slowing the evolution of FLD and avoiding its related consequences, such as liver cirrhosis and hepatocellular cancer. Lifestyle changes, such as eating a balanced diet, getting regular exercise, and avoiding excessive alcohol use, are critical in controlling FLD, especially in its non-alcoholic version.

Furthermore, the involvement of pharmacological treatments, such as insulin-sensitizing drugs and lipid-lowering pharmaceuticals, demonstrates the possibility of tailored therapy in certain patients of FLD. However, more research is needed to optimize treatment strategies and develop new therapeutic modalities that address the various underlying mechanisms of FLD.

The significance of raising awareness about FLD cannot be overstated, as early identification of risk factors and symptoms can lead to timely medical intervention and lifestyle changes. Healthcare providers play a critical role in educating patients about the importance of FLD and empowering them to make informed healthcare decisions.

Furthermore, addressing socioeconomic disparities and promoting equitable access to healthcare services are critical steps toward combating FLD on a larger scale. Public health initiatives aimed at lowering the prevalence of obesity, diabetes, and other metabolic disorders can help significantly prevent FLD and its complications.

In essence, FLD is a complex and multifaceted health challenge that necessitates a comprehensive and multidisciplinary strategy. By focusing on prevention, early detection, and tailored management strategies, we can work to reduce the burden of FLD and improve the overall health outcomes of those affected.

THE END

www.ingramcontent.com/pod-product-compliance
Lightning Source LLC
Chambersburg PA
CBHW070313230526
45470CB00002B/852